# KETO VEGAN

*Low Carb Diet Recipes For Weight Loss,*
*Fat Burning and Energy Boosting*
*Without A ton Of Effort*
*In the Next 7 days*

Holly R.Evans

# TABLE OF CONTENTS

**PART ONE: THE KETO-VEGAN LIFESTYLE**



**PART TWO: THE 7-DAY MEAL PLAN**



**PART THREE: PUTTING IT ALL TOGETHER**

**BREAKFAST**



**LUNCH**

# PART FOUR: CONCLUSION

# INTRODUCTION

The keto-vegan diet is a food guideline that comprises of low carbohydrates, moderate protein content and are rich in fats and oils. It became very popular over the years because of its tremendous efficiency on weight loss programs and general wellbeing. While the parent keto diet often has to do with animal foods, keto-vegan is based primarily on plant foods while still maintaining the original macro content ratios. Pure vegan diets is devoid of any animal product and as a result, it becomes increasingly difficult to consume low carbohydrate. The good news is, with careful planning of keto-vegan meals, vegans can as well benefit from the health promoting effects of a ketogenic diets. This work succinctly explains not just what to include and what to avoid in a well-planned ketogenic diet, it can also serve as a complete guide to anyone willing to adopt the keto-vegan dietary program and also provides a 7 days keto-vegan meal plan and recipes.

# PART ONE

## THE KETO-VEGAN LIFESTYLE

# CHAPTER 1

## Keto-vegan Diet Guide:

The keto-vegan diet is a food guideline that comprises of low carbohydrates, moderate protein content and are rich in fats and oils. It became very popular over the years because of its tremendous efficiency on weight loss programs and general wellbeing. While the parent keto diet often has to do with animal foods, keto-vegan is based primarily on plant foods while still maintaining the original macro content ratios. Pure vegan diets is devoid of any animal product and as a result, it becomes increasingly difficult to consume low carbohydrate. The good news is, with careful planning of keto-vegan meals, vegans can as well benefit from the health promoting effects of a ketogenic diets. This work succinctly explains not just what to include and what to avoid in a well-planned ketogenic diet, it can also serve as a complete guide to anyone willing to adopt the keto-vegan dietary program and also provides a 7 days keto-vegan meal plan and recipes.

## What Is the Keto-vegan Diet?

The keto-vegan diet comprises of foods that are low in carbohydrate content, contains moderate amounts of protein and are very rich (up to 80%) in fats and oils. In a typical keto-vegan meal, carbohydrates are drastically reduced to not even up to 50 grams per day. This is to enable the body reach and maintain a metabolic state called KETOSIS which is the goal of every ketogenic diet. Due to the fact that this dietary guideline is basically made of fats for the most part – somewhere around 80% of whole food – keto-vegans turn to high-oil plant products like avocado, olive, and coconut, making it possible for vegans, to also follow a ketogenic dietary guideline as well.

**The keto-Vegan diet comprises of moderate protein content, low carbohydrate, and is rich in fats and does not include any food of animal origin but plants.**

People on a vegan dietary guideline only take in food products of plant origin like grains, vegetables, and fruits and avoid any food of animal product like dairy, meats and poultry. Vegans are able to achieve and maintaining ketosis by subsisting on plant-based foods that are rich in fats content such as olive oil, coconut oil and avocados.

**WHY LOW-CARB, HIGH-FAT?**

EATING A HIGH FAT, LOW-CARBOHYDRATE DIET is important for every weight loss campaign. Even more importantly, findings from an increasing number of empirical researches shows that high-fat, low-carb foods help reduce an individual's chances and risks of coming down with systemic illnesses like heart disorders, diabetes, stroke or apoplexy, epilepsy and Alzheimer's. The keto-vegan dietary guideline promotes the consumption of fresh, organic whole foods like vegetables and fruits, and nourishing oils of plant origin. It's a dietary guideline with a long-term sustainability potential and is also enjoyable.

**Carbohydrates (sugar) brings about blood glucose sky-rocketing, which leads to crashes almost immediately, and then the accompanying cravings for more carbohydrates and sugars. This dangerous cascade of events leads to consistent spikes in insulin and the accompanying pre-diabetes and diabetes type II.**

Research findings consistently indicate that keto-vegan dietary guidelines enable people lose more pounds, causes improved energy levels for daily activities, curbs cravings and promotes long durations of satiety. The ability to curb cravings and promote satiety for long durations is because most of the caloric content in a keto-vegan diet originates from fat which is calorically dense and is slow in digestion. This makes it typical for keto-vegan eaters to consume lesser calories.

# CHAPTER 2

**Why Go Keto-Vegan?**

Consuming and maintaining a keto-vegan diet turns your body into an efficient machine for burning fat for metabolic fuel or energy. This is actually fantastic for a good number of reasons, not just that fats contains 2 times as much calories as carbohydrates, making you eat twice as less food by weight every day, the body attains a better position to get rid of stored fats (which a lot of people try so hard to burn) resulting in loss of more pounds. Making use of fats as a substrate for metabolic fuel ensures a consistent energy level for daily activities and the good news is, it does not mess with the blood glucose levels, thus with keto-vegan diets, you don't have to experience the lows and lows associated with consuming carbohydrates in high amounts. Consistent energy levels for the whole day means you can achieve more and as a matter of fact, feel less tired doing more.

In addition to the benefits highlighted above, consuming and maintaining keto-vegan diets for long can:

- Maintain steady levels of HDL (good) and LDL (bad) cholesterol
- Bring about more weight loss (specifically body fat)
- Decrease blood sugar and insulin resistance
- Improve brain function
- Decrease triglyceride levels
- Decrease blood pressure

## SUPPORT FOR YOUR NEW LIFESTYLE

When commencing the keto-vegan dietary program, it's very vital to let your family and closest friends or workplace colleagues to know you mean business concerning your new way of life and also detail them on the foods you need to stop eating. This has been proven to add strength to your support system as you will find helpful during social outings and gatherings like dinner and the rest. It's absolutely normal to be met with some resistance and challenges on start-up. Keep in mind that the high-fat, low-carb dietary guidelines has been the living standard in the lives of many people and keto-vegan is a complete turn of events. Just focus on yourself and the lifestyle goals you want to achieve. Sooner than you'll realize, your low levels of energy, reduction in body weight, and improved outlook will leave even naysayers wondering.

**One awesome place where you can start building your support system is reddit.com's keto-vegan sub reddit: www.reddit.com/r/keto-vegan**

**You'll discover numerous other keto-veganers from all around the globe sharing their experiences and progress notes, and also supporting others in this journey of complete turnaround.**

## Getting into Ketosis

When you are consuming and maintaining a diet that's rich in carbohydrate, your body is in a metabolic status known as glycolysis (sugar breakdown). The simple implication is that most of the metabolic fuel or energy your body uses for daily activities originates from blood glucose content. In this condition, immediately after each meal consumption, your blood glucose is sharply increased bringing about lower body insulin levels, and ths shortage in insulin drives the storage of body fat and also inhibits or prevents the release of fats from their storage sites (adipose tissues) in the body.

However, when you consume and maintain a low-carbohydrate, high-fat diet, the reverse becomes the case. Your body attains a metabolic condition known as KETOSIS. In this status, your body readily and efficiently breaks down fat into ketone bodies (ketones) for metabolic fuel as its primary energy source and fats storage sites are consistently emptied. It's a biologically normal state and you're not overriding anything as naysayers may think—as a matter of fact, whenever you consume low carbohydrate than your body requires, your body falls back to this status naturally.

## WHAT TO DO IF YOU HAVE DIABETES

The good news for persons with type 2 diabetes is that the keto-vegan low-carb, high-fat foods can start to kick in the diabetes condition in reverse gear. For type 1 diabetes, keto b-vegan can tremendously improve the body's control of blood glucose levels. Be sure to seek the counsel of your physician before embarking on any dietary guideline especially one that has to do with low carbohydrates intake. This is because if you take medications for diabetes type 1 for instance and want to embark on a low carbohydrate diet, it may become necessary and appropriate to reduce your dosages immediately. Your physician may recommend or suggest you embark on a period of trial or probation with your dietary guideline while he/she supervises. By so doing, they can maintain a close supervision on your blood glucose levels and insulin dosages. In addition, it is advisable to consume more than 50 grams of carbohydrate every day to prevent ketoacidosis in type 1 diabetes.

## TESTING FOR KETOSIS

As soon as you commence your low-carb keto-vegan diet, one thing you should know is when and if you have achieved the state of ketosis. Not only does it help in increasing your confidence levels on the journey, testing your ketosis status helps you know you're on the right track and whether there's need to make some changes. One very simple and easy test for ketosis is to sniff for "keto-breath." Few days from the moment you started eating low carb, it's normal for you to a fruity, metallic or even sour taste in your taste buds. This is because as soon as your body attains the state of ketosis, ketone bodies which are beta-hydroxybutyrate, acetoacetate and acetone are created in the body. Acetone is responsible for ketone breathe as it is excreted from the breath and the urine. Also, ketone urine test strips are also used to more accurately detect the presence of ketone bodies (acetone).

Similar to the USDA's Food Pyramid, the keto-vegan dietary guidelines is developed on macro ratios. It's very essential to obtain the appropriate macronutrients so as not to deprive your body of the energy it requires for daily activities and also of any essential dietary fat or protein. Macronutrients are carbohydrates, proteins and fats and are the major building blocks of the food we eat. Each one of the macros provides the body with a given amount of metabolic fuel or energy measure in calories per gram of macro eaten.

- **Fat = 9 calories per gram**
- **Protein = 4 calories per gram**
- **Carbohydrates = 4 calories per gram**

With the keto-vegan dietary guideline, about 75% percent of the calories intake is expected to be obtained from oils, while about 20 % is obtained from plant-based protein foods and the last 5% from carbohydrate foods of plant origin.

**The number of calories you should eat depends on a few factors, including:**

- **Current lean body weight**
- **The types of workouts**
- **Hours per week of each type**
- **Daily activity levels**
- **Gain muscle**
- **Maintain weight**
- **Workout regimen? If so:**
- **Goals**
- **Lose weight**

You can also find plenty of helpful tools for calculation with a quick Google search for "keto calculator." You'll be able to easily and quickly plug in your numbers and get an immediate estimation of your body's caloric needs.

One of the great things about the keto diet is that it's not necessary to track each and every number to hit your goals. Yet if you want to track, it's a great way to speed up your progress, and tracking will give you a visual reminder to stay on course every day.

**Necessary Nutrients**

It's crucial to drink plenty of water when beginning the keto-vegan diet. In addition, it is also absolutely normal for you to be visiting the convenience more often. This happens because since you're drastically reducing your intake of processed or refined foods and have started eating organic and natural food products, you're also reducing your intake of certain minerals like sodium which is found in refined or processed foods so the abrupt dietary modification causes a sudden low in sodium intake.

More so, the sudden decrease in carbohydrate intake also reduces the level of insulin in the body, making the kidneys to release more sodium. As a result, the body removes more water through urine, causing you to urinate often and lose water and electrolytes.

When this is the case, the typical symptoms includes headaches, fatigue, nausea, and irritability.

**This state is for the most part known as the "keto flu." It's imperative to realize this isn't the real influenza virus. It's known as the keto flu just because of the likeness in symptoms, however it's neither infectious nor a genuine virus.**

Numerous people who encounter these symptoms trust the keto diet made them wiped out and promptly return to eating carbs. In any case, the keto flu stage really implies your body is pulling back from sugar, high carbs, and refined foods, and is straightening out so it can utilize fat as its fuel. The keto flu as a rule keeps going only a couple of days while the body rearranges. You can lessen its symptoms by adding more sodium and electrolytes to your eating regimen.

## THE "KETO FLU"

The keto flu is avoidable and its duration can be reduced simply by adding more sodium to your diet. Here are some of the easiest ways to do it:

- Add more salt to your meals.
- Eat saltier foods like pickled vegetables and bacon.

## Keto-vegan Weight Loss basics for Biggest Losers

1. **Check Out What Shape You're In**

   Start with a health check. See your GP and check out what shape your health is in, including blood pressure, cholesterol and blood sugar levels. Check your starting weight, waist and hip measurements. Write them down in a journal.

2. **Set A Weight Loss Goal**

   Start off by aiming to lose 5-10% of your starting weight. If you weigh 100 kilograms, aim to get to 90 kilograms over three to six months. Most people are not aware that losing this amoint of weight will reduce their risk of developing type 2 diabetes and greatly improve their health. Plus, it is a realistic goal.

3. **Get Organized**

   Get organized for a healthy Keto-vegan eating. This means you need to have a clean-up day in your kitchen! Get rid of all the junk foods and drinks lurking around in the panty, freezer and any secret hiding spot. Successful keto-vegan biggest losers plan their meal ahead of time. Plan out a whole week of meals in advance and then write out a matching grocery list. Do not buy foods that are not on the list or foods that do not belong there in a successful keto-vegan biggest loser's pantry, fridge or freezer.

4.  **Make A Hobby Out Of Reading Food Labels.**
    Use the recipe and meal plan guide in this book to make over for your recipes in the keto-vegan biggest loser's style.

5.  **Eat Your Way To Weight-Loss Healthy Living Success**
    Low carb, high fat meals turn keto-vegan biggest losers into weight loss winners. This means dramatically increasing your low carb vegetables, salads and fruits intake and also using the various forms of meat alternatives out there. Try a home delivery of fruits and vegetables service so that big quantities arrive automatically and give you an extra incentive to us emore of them. Plus it can be cheaper and the produce is delivered straight from the markets.

6. **Keep A Record Of What You Eat And How Active You Are**

   Every day, record what you eat and drink, as well as the physical activities and exercises you do. Use this information to work out which foods that provide most of your Calories and fat over bthe day. This is called self-monitoring. It keeps you honest about what you eat, ensuring you abide by the keto-vegan Do's and Don'ts. It also shows you how much exercise it will take to burn off your favorite treats and highlights how easily extra calories can sneak into your day.

## Getting Ready to Go Keto-Vegan

Now that you understand the benefits and science behind the keto-vegan diet, you're ready to get started. In the following chapters, you'll get all the information you need to succeed with your keto-vegan diet, including what to buy and what to avoid, meal plans and full recipes, and physical activities or exercises to carry out to be in top health.

# CHAPTER 3

**GO KETO-VEGAN IN FIVE STEPS**

Now that you've known the facts behind the low-carb high-fat keto-vegan dietary guidelines and why it does what you're about to experience. In this section, you'll figure out how to begin and amplify achievement. Here's a snappy and simple well-ordered manual for use as you start, and to allude to whenever all through your adventure, for help and direction.

## Step 1: Clean Out Your Pantry

Out with the old, in with the new. Having tempting, unhealthy foods in your home is one of the biggest contributors to failure when starting any diet. To succeed, you need to minimize any triggers to maximize your chances. Unless you have the iron will of Arnold Schwarzenegger, you should not keep addictive foods like bread, desserts, and other non–keto friendly snacks around.

If you don't live alone, be sure to discuss and warn your housemates, whether they're significant others, family, or roommates. If some items must be kept (if they're simply not yours to throw out), try to agree on a special location to keep them out of sight. This will also help anyone you share your living space with understand that you are serious about starting your diet, and will lead to a better experience for you at home overall (people love to tempt anyone on a diet at first, but it will get old and they'll tire quickly).

## STARCHES AND GRAINS

Do away with all high carbohydrate food like pasta, rice, potatoes, bread, corns, bagels, oats, and croissants.

## SUGARY FOODS AND DRINKS

Do away with all refined sugar foods and drinks like fruit juices, fountain drinks, fruit juices, pastries, candy bars, etc.

## LEGUMES

Do away with beans, lentils, and peas. They are rich in carbohydrate contents. A 1-cup serving of beans alone provides more than triple of your daily carbohydrate allowance on a low-carb high-fat diet.

## PROCESSED POLYUNSATURATED FATS AND OILS

Get rid of all vegetable oils and most seed oils, including sunflower, safflower, canola, soybean, grapeseed, and corn oil.

Also eliminate trans fats like shortening and margarine—anything that says "hydrogenated" or "partially hydrogenated." Olive oil, extra-virgin olive oil, avocado oil, and coconut oil are the keto-vegan-friendly oils you want on hand.

**FRUITS**

Get rid of fruits that are high in carbs, including bananas, dates, grapes, mangos, and apples. Be sure to get rid of any dried fruits like raisins as well. Dried fruit contains as much sugar as regular fruit but more concentrated, making it easy to eat a lot of sugar in a small serving. For comparison, a cup of raisins has over 100 grams of carbs while a cup of grapes has only 15 grams of carbs.

Yes, you're "getting rid" of unwanted foods in your pantry, but these foods can feed many others. Please, don't throw them away! Find a local food bank or homeless youth shelter to donate them to.Your pantry will seem empty after the cleanout. That's because products meant for longer-term storage are usually high in carbs and full of unhealthy additives and preservatives. You'll fill your refrigerator shortly (Step 2) with healthy, natural foods.

**FINDING SUPPORT**

Sticking to your diet in the beginning can prove difficult when close friends and family aren't eating the same as you. Even worse, they are eating all the things you're trying not to eat. Every person is different, and you likely know who will support you and who will not. For those who support you, explain that you're avoiding carbs (and which foods include carbs) and request politely that they not offer you anything when you're eating together.

Telling the naysayers that you've quit eating grains and sugar will usually suffice. The terms keto-vegan and low-carb will usually spark a debate or argument with certain people because they've been told their whole lives to eat carbs and low-fat products. Try to avoid using those terms when explaining your diet goals. Avoid direct debates by recommending they read about the benefits of being in ketosis and the health benefits of eating a low-carb diet.

## Step 2: Go Shopping

It's time to restock your pantry, refrigerator, and freezer with delicious, keto-friendly foods that will help you lose weight, become healthy, and feel great!

### VEGGIES

You can eat all no starchy veggies, including broccoli, asparagus, mushrooms, cucumbers, lettuce, onions, peppers, tomatoes, garlic (in small quantities—each clove contains about 1 gram of carbs), Brussels sprouts, zucchini, eggplant, olives, zucchini, yellow squash, and cauliflower.

Avoid all types of potatoes, yams and sweet potatoes, corn, and legumes like beans, lentils, and peas.

### SWEETENERS ...

The sweeteners may sound strange if you haven't heard of them before. They both come from natural sources and are safe to use in any quantity. Stevia is naturally obtained from the leaves of a plant by name Stevia rebaudiana. Stevia has zero calories and contains some beneficial micronutrients like magnesium, potassium, and zinc. It's readily available in liquid or powder form online and in most supermarkets. It's much sweeter than sugar, so containers are usually very small—you won't need nearly as much. Erythritol is a sugar alcohol that is low in calories, about 70 percent as sweet as sugar, and can be found naturally in some fruits and vegetables. Sugar alcohols are indigestible by the human body, so erythritol cannot raise your blood sugar or insulin levels. Several studies have proven it to be safe. Sugar alcohols can sometimes cause temporary digestive discomfort, but out of the few available sugar alcohols like xylitol, maltitol, and sorbitol, erythritol is considered to be the most forgiving and best for everyday use.

## FRUITS

You can eat a small amount of berries every day, such as strawberries, raspberries, blackberries, and blueberries. Lemon and lime juices are great for adding flavor to your meals. Avocados are also low in carbs and full of healthy fat. Avoid other fruits, as they're loaded with sugar. A single banana can contain around 25 grams of net carbs.

## DAIRY ALTERNATIVES

Although not technically dairy, unsweetened almond and coconut milks are great alternatives for keto-vegan diets as well. Avoid milk and skim milk, as well as sweetened yogurt, as it contains a lot of sugar. Avoid any flavored, low-fat, or fat-free dairy products.

**FATS AND OILS**

Avocado oil, olive oil, butter, lard, and bacon fat are great for cooking and consuming. Avocado oil has a high smoke point (it does not burn or smoke until it reaches 520°F), which is ideal for searing meats and frying in a wok. Make sure to avoid oils labeled "blend"; they commonly contain small amounts of the healthy oil and large amounts of unhealthy oils.

## Step 3: Set Up Your Kitchen

Preparing delicious recipes is one of the best parts of the keto-vegan diet, and it's quite easy if you have the right tools. The following tools will make cooking simpler and faster. Each one is worth investing in, especially for the busy cook.

**FOOD SCALE**

When you're trying to hit your caloric and macronutrient goals, a kitchen food scale is a necessary appliance. You can measure any solid or liquid food, and get the perfect amount every time. Used in combination with an app like MyFitnessPal, you'll have all the data you need to hit your goals sooner. Food scales can be found online for $10 to $20.

**FOOD PROCESSOR**

Food processors are critical to your arsenal. They are ideal for blending certain foods or processing foods together into sauces and shakes. Blenders don't cut it, powerwise, for many foods, especially tough vegetables like cauliflower. One great food processor/blender is

NutriBullet. The containers you blend in come with lids or drink spouts so you can take them to go or use them as storage. They're also easy to clean, making the whole system extremely convenient. They typically sell for about $80 online.

## SPIRALIZER

Spiralizers make vegetables into noodles or ribbons within seconds. They make cooking a lot faster and easier—noodles have much more surface area and take a fraction of the time to cook. For example, a spiralizer turns a zucchini into noodles, and with some Alfredo or marinara sauce, you can't tell you aren't eating noodles. Spiralizers cost around $30 and can be found in large retail stores and online.

## ELECTRIC HAND MIXER

If you've ever had to beat an egg white by hand until you get stiff peaks, then you know just how difficult it is. Electric hand mixers save your arm muscles and massive amounts of time, especially when mixing heavy ingredients. You can find a decent one online for $10 to $20.

## CAST IRON PANS

They've been used for centuries and were one of the first modern cooking devices. Cast iron skillets don't wear out and are healthier to use (no chemical treatment of any kind), retain heat very well, and can be moved between the stove and oven. They are simple to clean up—just wash them out with a scrub sponge without soap, dry them off, and then rub them with cooking oil. This prevents rust and encourages the

buildup of "seasoning," a natural nonstick surface. Many cast iron pans come pre-seasoned, and this method preserves the coating. You can find them in many retail stores and online for $10 to $80, depending on the brand and size; Lodge is a popular brand, still made in the United States.

## KNIFE SHARPENING STONE

Most of prep time is spent on cutting. You'll see your cutting speed skyrocket with a sharp knife set. It's also a pleasure to use sharp knives. Aim to sharpen your knives every week or so to keep them in good shape (professional chefs sharpen their knives before every use). Sharpening stones cost under $10 and can be ordered online.

## NICE-TO-HAVE EQUIPMENT

The kitchen section of any store can be a wonderland. There are so many intriguing gadgets. It's also nice (although not necessary) to have these other tools on hand if you can't resist the lure:

## INSTANT COOKING THERMOMETER

Cooking steak and chicken is much easier when you can easily prod the meat and find out whether it's at the level of doneness that you're shooting for. These can usually be found for $10 to $20 in most retail stores or online.

**MEASURING SPOON SET**

Get the right amount of an ingredient quickly. These sets can go from $5 to $10 in any supermarket, store, or online.

**TONGS**

Tongs reduce splatter when working quickly (compared to using a fork or spatula to flip something in a hot pan). It's best to get tongs with nylon heads so you don't scratch any of your pots or pans. You can get a pair online or in retail stores for $10 to $15.

## Step 4: Meal Plan

Using meal plans in the beginning of your diet greatly increases your chances of success. The meal plans in part 2 of this book include meals for every part of the day, premade shopping lists, and macronutrient and calorie counts for each meal. They even account for leftovers. This will make starting out much easier and more enjoyable!

**Meal plans work well because they give you goals and direction. If you know what you need to make next without thinking about it, you're less likely to give up, change your mind, and order food from your favorite takeout spot. Also, since you know what's coming next, you can look forward to it throughout the day and week.**

Pay attention to the ingredients listed on the packaged products you buy. The best products have just a few ingredients with recognizable names, meaning they're made with fewer additives and preservatives.

After using the meal plans for a few weeks, you set your body up to have the right expectations for how much food you'll provide it and what type of food it will get (high in fat and protein and low in carbs). Even if you don't continue to use meal plans, you'll be familiar enough with the diet to know what you should be eating and how much.

## Step 5: Exercise

As you start your diet and the pounds fall off, think about how to lose more weight or get healthier to feel even better.

This is a great time to become more active through exercise.

Increase the amount you exercise relative to what you do now. If you don't exercise at all, start taking short walks or slow jogs, or a combination of both, for 15 minutes every other day. If you already go to the gym or lift weights, add an extra exercise or start doing cardio. It doesn't matter what level you're at, try to do a little more than you're doing now. That's all it takes to become healthier. Exercise is incremental, and every increment is a boost to weight loss and feeling better.

If you have the time, try taking a class or doing an activity that involves moving, like a step class or dancing, or start playing a sport like basketball. It doesn't have to be competitive, nor do you need to be good or have any previous experience. Such activities are an easy way to get on your feet, and you can learn a new skill in the process.

Staying fit through regular physical activity has been proven to reduce blood pressure and cholesterol levels as well as reduce risk for various heart diseases and type 2 diabetes. In combination with the keto diet, your health will improve dramatically, and so will your energy levels. Any exercise, even if it's 15 minutes a week, is better than no exercise. Don't worry about how much you do in the beginning. Just start doing something and you'll build from there naturally.

## EASY EXERCISE SEQUENCES

Here are a few easy exercise sequences if you're just starting out. Once every other day is enough in the beginning. If possible, try doing these with a friend or significant other for support and accountability. If you can't do some of them, that's absolutely all right! Simply focus on the ones you can do.

## CARDIOVASCULAR ACTIVITY

Any aerobic activity, like walking, running, or bicycling, for 15 to 30 minutes, twice a week or more.

## STRENGTH CONDITIONING

One set of exercises (for at least 10 repetitions, or it's too easy) targeting each of the major muscle groups: chest, shoulders, back, abs, and legs.

- Push-ups or assisted push-ups
- Pull-ups or chin-ups
- Crunches
- Squats

# PART TWO

## THE 7 DAYS MEAL PLAN AND RECIPES

# CHAPTER 4

## THE 7 DAYS MEAL PLAN

Here comes the long awaited 7 Day Keto-vegan Diet Plan! The caloric count of each day in this meal plan is set at 1600-1750 calories. However, if there is need for an increment, you can add more oils by lightly drizzling them over your meal or you can as well try adding one tablespoon of coconut oil to your coffee.

| | MONDAY | TUESDAY | WEDNESDAY | THURSDAY | FRIDAY | SATURDAY | SUNDAY |
|---|---|---|---|---|---|---|---|
| BREAKFAST | Blackberry Coconut Breakfast Bowl | Blackberry Coconut Breakfast Bowl | Chocolate Raspberry Chia Pudding Shots | Curry Tofu Scramble with Avocado | Chocolate Raspberry Chia Pudding Shots | Curry Tofu Scramble with Avocado | Curry Tofu Scramble with Avocado |
| LUNCH | Chia Flaxseed crackers with Guacamole | Chia Flaxseed crackers with Guacamole | Garlic Brocolli on Cauliflower Rice | Garlic Brocolli on Cauliflower Rice | Asian Sesame Tofu Salad | Asian Sesame Tofu Salad | Asian Sesame Tofu Salad |
| DINNER | Almond Coconut Curry on Veges | Almond Coconut Curry on Veges | Tofu Spinach Curry (Saag Paneer) | Tofu Spinach Curry (Saag Paneer) | Tofu Spinach Curry (Saag Paneer) | Spinach, Avocado and Pumpkin Seed Salad | Spinach, Avocado and Pumpkin Seed Salad |

| | | | | | | | |
|---|---|---|---|---|---|---|---|
| **DAILY SNACKS** | 1 1/2 oz almonds Mocha Protein Shake (No coconut oil) | 1 1/2 oz almonds Vanilla Protein Shake (No coconut oil) | 1 1/2 oz almonds Chocolate Protein Shake (1/8 cup coconut oil) | 1/2 oz almonds Mocha Protein Shake (1/8 cup coconut oil) | 1 1/2 oz almonds Vanilla Protein Shake (1/8 cup coconut oil) | Chocolate Protein Shake (1/8 cup coconut oil) | Mocha Protein Shake (1/8 cup coconut oil) |
| **DESSERTS** | Pumpkin Spice Fat Bombs | Pumpkin Spice Fat Bombs | Blueberry Fat Bombs | Spiced-Chocolate Fat Bombs | Chocolate-Coconut Treats | Almond Butter Fudge | Peanut Butter Mousse |
| **TOTAL CALORIES** | Calories (kcal): 1636 Fats(g): 130 Protein(g): 71 Net Carbs(g): 29.5 | Calories (kcal): 1626 Fats(g): 130 Protein(g): 71 Net Carbs(g): 29.5 | Calories (kcal): 1652 Fats(g): 137 Protein(g): 68 Net Carbs(g): 28.5 | Calories (kcal): 1710 Fats(g): 142 Protein(g): 72 Net Carbs(g): 29.5 | Calories (kcal): 1725 Fats(g): 140 Protein(g): 76 Net Carbs(g): 29.5 | Calories (kcal): 1611 Fats(g): 132 Protein(g): 67 Net Carbs(g): 25.0 | Calories (kcal): 1611 Fats(g): 132 Protein(g): 67 Net Carbs(g): 25.0 |

## Planning Ahead:

Once your kitchen is organized for cooking, the next step is to plan an approximate weekly keto-vegan menu. Do this by writing out what meals you would like to cook for the next week. Do these BEFORE you do your grocery shopping. To make life a little easier on your busy nights, aim to cook meals that are fast to assemble. Plan one night where you can cook a double quantity of your recipe so you can reheat the leftovers for another night. On the weekend, try making two dishes and refrigerated one. Then give yourself a night off during the weekend.

Once you've written down this meal plan this way, create a shopping list to match it. Check your fridge or freezer and pantry to see which ingredients you already have. Go for grocery shopping after you have had a meal so you are not tempted to purchase a meal not on your list.

Keep your meal plan on the fridge or any other conspicuous place in the kitchen. When you arrive tired and hungry at the end of the day you will be really pleased to see the hard work of deciding "what's for dinner" is done. You will also discover you start to prepare dinner on auto-pilot mode.

**ADDITIONAL TIPS**
- **Aim for 1200-1500 calories per day, as a minimum intake to ensure you get all the nutrients you need form food to keep you healthy while you are losing weight.**
- **The ideal rate of weight loss is ½ to 1 kilogram of body weight per day.**
- **You may lose weight faster in the first few weeks due to changes in energy and water storage.**
- **If you lose weight faster than 1 kilo per week after the first few weeks, you can increase your average daily calorie intake.**

There are many facets to following a healthy lifestyle, but healthy eating should be at the top of the list. Finding time to plan meals is the greatest route to proper eating and healthy living and it starts with being able to know which foods to pick up from the grocery store and preparing the foods in such a way you will enjoy daily. These comes with some challenges to anyone who wants to plan and pattern meals in a way to feel energized and maintain or lose weight and feel energized as nothing good comes easy.. Many of us have full time jobs with aging parents to take care of; children and other responsibilities making us have busy schedules with little or no time for ourselves.  The goal of this article is to outline some important meal planning challenges and point out the best ways to overcome them so you can eat right and live healthy.

Here is the most common meal planning challenges and their solutions or means to overcome them


1.    Healthy meals take much time to prepare
Solution:
Utilize precut vegetables and other healthy convenient foods. Search for crisp onions, celery, carrots, chime peppers, broccoli, cauliflower, and mushrooms sold in the deliver path. Likewise use pre-marinated lean meats, rotisserie-cooked chicken bosoms, quartered marinated artichokes, preminced garlic and ginger, and canned beans, canned fish, and shredded reduced-fat cheddar to spare prep time.

2.    The kids usually have their separate meals and can hardly fit into the plan.

Solution:

Prepare 1 diet yet season it in 2 diverse ways. For example, on pasta night, make a striking tasting sauce for the grown-ups, but warm up bumped spaghetti sauce for the children. When making meals, partition the blend fifty-fifty, enhance every half in a different way, at that point fill the two sides of the meal dish and stamp them with toothpicks so you'll know which will be which.

3.      We often eat in restaurants and  take some food home

Solution

Reduce eating out or takeout suppers to once or at most two times every week. Rather than creamy or fried dishes, place order for dishes that are heated, cooked, barbecued, or steamed. Request that sauces and dressing be served by the side of your order. If your food does not contain enough vegetables, request an additional serving.

4.  Majority of our planned healthy meals don't really taste great.

Solution:

Tape a chart of herbs/flavors and their matching foods inside your pantry for simple reference. For instance, thyme runs well with chicken and mushrooms and rosemary with lean meat. Include seasoning with sun-dried tomatoes, hot pepper sauce, balsamic vinegar, and salsa or lemon juice for an additional lift.

# PART THREE

## PUTTING ALL RECIPES TOGETHER

# Delicious Keto-Vegan Food Lists

**BREAKFAST**

1. Chocolate-Raspberry Chia Pudding Shots
2. Curry Tofu Scramble with Avocado
3. Blackberry Coconut Breakfast Bowl

**DINNER**

4. Almond Coconut Curry on Veges
5. Tofu Spinach Curry (Saag Paneer)
6. Spinach, Avocado and Pumpkin Seed Salad

**LUNCH**

7. Garlic Broccoli on Cauliflower Rice
8. Asian Sesame Tofu Salad
9. Chia Flaxseed Crackers with Guacamole

**DAILY SNACKS**

10. Keto Chocolate Protein Shake (Part 1)
11. Keto Chocolate Protein Shake (Part 2)
12. Keto Vanilla Protein Shake

**DESSERTS**

13. Pumpkin Spice Fat Bombs
14. Blueberry Fat Bombs
15. Spiced-Chocolate Fat Bombs
16. Chocolate-Coconut Treats
17. Almond Butter Fudge
18. Peanut Butter Mousse

# BREAKFAST

# Chocolate-Raspberry Chia Pudding Shots

Dessert and breakfast, together once more! These Chocolate-Raspberry Chia pudding shots are relatively similar to enchantment. They're solid and sweet - the ideal mix. Celebrated for being a low carb thickening agent, these natural chia seeds make a remarkable pudding!

Course: Breakfast, Dessert;
Prep Time 1 hour;
Servings 2; Calories 240 kcal

## INGREDIENTS:

- ¼ cup chia seeds

- 1/2 cup coconut milk

- 1/4 cup almond milk

- 1 tablespoon cacao powder

- 1 tablespoon Stevia

- 1/2 cup raspberries

1. In a container, bring together all the ingredients (with the exception of the raspberries) and shake vivaciously. Let sit for 2 minutes and after that fill four shot glasses.

2. Refrigerate for no less than 60 minutes (ideally across the night) until the point that blend thickens into pudding. Top with raspberries.

**Recipe Notes:**

**This yield of this recipe is 4 shots. 1 serving is 2 shots.**

**Nutritional Information:**

Calories: 241, Protein: 4g Fats: 20g, , Net Carbs: 4g

# Curry Tofu Scramble with Avocado

This tofu scramble is a fabulous low carb veggie lover approach to
begin the morning, with a lot of supplements and sufficient calories to
give you vitality for the day ahead.


Course: Breakfast;
Prep Time 5 minutes;
Total Time 20 minutes, Cook Time 13 minutes; Calories 380 kcal Servings 3

## INGREDIENTS:

- 1 tbsp coconut oil

- 2 tbsp olive oil

- 300 g tofu (extra firm)

- 1 tsp turmeric

- 1 tbsp nutritional yeast

- 1 tbsp curry powder

- 1/2 cup zucchini (chopped)

- 1 cup mushrooms (chopped)

- 1 tomato (chopped)

- cilantro (optional)(to garnish)

- 300-gram avocado

# INSTRUCTIONS:

- The initial step is to dry the tofu so it ingests the flavor.
- Cut the tofu into 1 inch long strips, spread out the strips on a paper towel,
- put another paper towel to finish everything and after that a slashing board.
- Place something substantial over this, for example, a few books.
- Abandon it to sit for around 15 minutes.
- Add the coconut oil to the dish and disintegrate the tofu into the skillet with your hands.
- Cook for around 5 minutes, mixing every now and again.
- Include the turmeric, nourishing yeast and curry powder and 1 tbsp of the olive oil,
- blend and cook for a further 4 minutes.
- Add whatever remains of the olive oil, zucchini, mushroom and tomato and sear for a further 4 minutes blending much of the time.
- Serve with 1 little medium size avocado (roughly 100g) cut.

**Recipe Notes:**

**This meal can be refrigerated for a few days.**

**Nutritional Information:**

Calories: 381, Fats: 32g, Protein: 11g, Net Carbs: 8g

# Blackberry Coconut Breakfast Bowl

This breakfast bowl is smooth and rich, and has the magnificent FLAVORS of blackberry and coconut. An extraordinary begin to the day. It's likewise super simple and snappy to get ready!

Course Breakfast;
Total Time 5 minutes; Prep Time 5 minutes; Calories 467 kcal ; Servings 2

## INGREDIENTS:

. 1 cup blackberries

. 1 cup coconut milk

. 3 tbsp ground flaxseed

. 1/4 cup water

. 1 cup spinach

. 1/4 cup coconut flakes

. 2 tbsp chia seeds

# INSTRUCTIONS:

1. Mix the flaxseed with the water in a glass until the point that the water is assimilated (just needs around 10 seconds).
2. Pour a large portion of the blackberries (sparing some for trimming), coconut drain, spinach and the flaxseed blend into a blender and mix until smooth.
3. In a different sear the coconut drops for a moment or two on high warmth to toast them.
4. Pour the berry blend into two dishes and sprinkle the rest of the ground flaxseed on top alongside the chia seeds and coconut pieces. Appreciate promptly.

**Recipe Notes:**
**You can store the blackberry blend in the ice chest and utilize it the following day in the event that you like. Note this formula makes two servings - the beneath dietary data is for one serving.**

**Nutritional Information:**

Calories: 465, Fats: 43g, Protein: 8g, Net Carbs: 7g

# LUNCH

# Asian Sesame Tofu Salad

This Asian Sesame Tofu Salad is delectable, flavorsome and truly keto! The tofu assimilates the flours rice vinegar, sesame and tamari, while the zucchini, cucumber and spinach serve to keep it feeling new. The pumpkin seeds additionally include a decent crunch.

Course Dinner, Lunch, Main Dish, Salad; Cuisine Japanese; Total Time 33 minutes; Prep Time 10 minutes; Cook Time 23 minutes; Calories 406 kcal Servings 3;

## INGREDIENTS:

**For the tofu:**
**For the salad:**

- **400 g tofu (1 packet, extra firm)**

- **4 cups spinach**

- **4 tbsp olive oil**

- **1 zucchini (sliced into thin strips)**

- **2 tsp tamari**

- **1 cucumber (chopped into semi circles)**

- **1 1/2 tsp sesame oil**

- **1 tsp ginger (crushed)**

- **2 tbsp rice vinegar**

- **1/4 cup sesame seeds**

- **1/4 cup pumpkin seeds**

**INSTRUCTIONS:**

1. Mix 3 tbsp olive oil and the majority of the tamari, sesame oil, ginger and rice vinegar together in a bowl.
2. Cut the tofu into 1 inch long strips and put into a skillet on medium high warmth. Include 1/2 of the dressing to the container and coat the tofu. Sear for around 10-15 minutes, precisely blending the pieces around in oil at regular intervals with a spatula until the point when the tofu is brilliant dark colored. Include the sesame seeds and 1/4 of the dressing to the dish and broil with the tofu for 2-3 minutes.
3. Add the zucchini and cucumber to the bowl with the rest of the 1/4 of the dressing. Mix precisely for around 5 minutes. Expel from the warmth.
4. Heat a little griddle at medium, include 1 tbsp of olive oil and the pumpkin seeds. Sear for a couple of minutes until toasted.
5. Serve the Asian tofu over crude spinach leaves, and best with toasted pumpkin seeds.

**Recipe Notes:**

**Stir the tofu with the oil carefully so as not to break.**

**Nutritional Information:**

Calories: 407, Fats: 34g, Protein: 14g, Net Carbs: 7g

# Garlic Broccoli on Cauliflower Rice

This meal is so basic and is a staple for us. The supplement thick broccoli and the light and completely cauliflower rice mix well with the kinds of garlic and oil.

Course Dinner, Lunch;
Prep Time 5 minutes; Cook Time 10 minutes;
Total Time 15 minutes;
Servings 2; Calories 323 kcal

## INGREDIENTS:

**For the Broccoli:**
> **For the cauliflower rice:**

- **1.5 cup broccoli (chopped into florets)**
- **1.5 cup Cauliflower (chopped into florets)**
- **3 tablespoons extra-virgin olive oil**
- **2 cloves garlic (crushed)**
- **1/2 cup pumpkin seeds**
- **1 tbsp lemon juice**
- **salt (to taste)**

## INSTRUCTIONS:

1. Put the cauliflower florets into a sustenance processor and heartbeat a couple of times until the point when it transforms into minor rice measured granules. Set aside.

2.  Place a dish on medium high warmth and pour in 1 tbsp of the olive oil, pounded garlic and pumpkin seeds. Warmth for a couple of minutes to toast the pumpkin seeds and discharge the kind of the garlic.
3.  Add the broccoli to the dish and panfry for around 5 minutes.
4.  Add the lemon squeeze and salt and panfry for an additional 2 minutes.
5.  Serve on promptly with the crude cauliflower rice and sprinkle 1 tbsp of olive oil over the highest point of each serving.

**Recipe Notes:**

**Don't hesitate to swap the broccoli out for other low carb vegetables. Now and then we'll cook 1/2 container mushrooms and 1/2 measure of zucchini with the supper instead of the asparagus. Eat an assortment of vegetables in your eating routine. Additionally be liberal with the garlic as it works as the essential flavor. In the event that you need to include/decrease the calories simply alter the additional olive oil. You can likewise swap out the pumpkin seeds for Hemp Seeds or another seed on the off chance that you like.**

**Nutritional Information:**

Calories: 322, Fats: 30g, Protein: 7g, Net Carbs: 8g

# Chia Flaxseed Crackers with Guacamole

These Chia Flaxseed Crackers make for an extraordinary dinner or tidbit. They're simple, cook rapidly and can be put away for utilize later in the week. An extraordinary keto-veggie lover feast.

Course Dinner, Lunch;
Cook Time 2 hours 20 minutes; Prep Time 25 minutes;
Total Time 2 hours 45 minutes;
Servings 4; Calories 256 kcal

## INGREDIENTS:

**For the guacamole**
    **For the crackers**

- **1 avocado**
- **35 g whole flaxseed**
- **1 small tomato (chopped into 1cm cubes)**
- **50 g ground flaxseed**
- **1 lime (juiced)**
- **40 g chia seeds**
- **1 garlic clove (small, crushed)**
- **1 tbsp tamari**
- **1 tbsp cilantro (chopped)**
- **1 pinch sea salt**
- **1 cup of water**

**INSTRUCTIONS:**

**For the avocado:**

1. Mix the majority of the fixings in a bowl utilizing a fork until the point that the coveted guacamole consistency is achieved.

## For the flax seed crackers:

1. Preheat the broiler to 140 degrees
2. Mix every one of the elements for the chia seed saltines in a bowl and let the blend thicken for 15 minutes.
3. Warm a broiler plate in the stove, expel the plate and line it with preparing paper. Press the blend onto the heating paper, spreading it equitably. Prepare for 1 hour 40 minutes or until fresh. You may need to alter the time contingent upon the broiler, yet it takes a reasonable while.
4. After 1 hour 40 minutes the wafer blend ought to be decent and firm. Presently flip the blend over, turn the broiler onto fan barbecue and leave in the stove for an additional 40 minutes to fresh up the underside. You can build the warmth here with the end goal to lessen the time required, however be mindful so as not to consume the blend.
5. Remove from the broiler and cut into 4 areas, with 2 saltines for every segment. Present with the guacamole and appreciate!

**Recipe Notes:**

**You can store the saltines in a sealed shut compartment in the pantry and essentially place them in the broiler for a fast 5 minutes before serving. Additionally take note of the picture we utilized for this completed formula is a twofold serving. You can have a couple of servings relying upon your caloric prerequisites.**

**Nutritional Information (One serving):**
Calories: 256, Fats: 19g, Protein: 7g, Net Carbs: 5g

# DINNER

# Almond Coconut Curry on Veges

 This almond coconut curry is super speedy and simple and tastes extraordinary as well! It flaunts nutritious vegetables alongside solid fats and a decent calorie tally.

Course Dinner, Lunch; Cook
Time 15 minutes; Total Time 15 minutes;
Servings 4; Calories 439 kcal

## INGREDIENTS:

**For the veges**
**For the curry**

- **1 tsp coconut oil**
- **400 ml coconut milk**
- **2 cups mushrooms**
- **125 g almond butter (100% ground almonds)**
- **4 cups spinach**
- **1 tbsp tomato paste**
- **2 cups brocolli (chopped into florets)**
- **1 tbsp curry powder**

## INSTRUCTIONS:
**For the curry mixture**

1. Put the coconut drain, almond spread, tomato glue and curry powder in a blender. Mix for around 20 seconds or until smooth.

2.  Add the curry blend to a pan on low-medium warmth and warmth for 10-15 minutes or until warmed through. Blend habitually to abstain from staying.

**For the veges**

1.  Heat the coconut oil in a container on medium-high warmth and include the broccoli and mushrooms. Sear for around 3 minutes. Include the spinach and warmth for one more moment.

2.  Serve the veges in a bowl with the curry blend poured over the best.

**Recipe Notes:**

**You can make the almond margarine by granulating almonds in a sustenance processor.**

**The curry blend isolates whenever left to sit in the refrigerator for some time, so make certain to mix it completely before utilizing on the off chance that you have put away it in the ice chest.**
**Nutritional Information:**

Calories: 438, Fats: 41g, Protein: 11g, Net Carbs: 9g

# Tofu Spinach Curry (Saag Paneer)

A delicious vegan keto take on an Indian classic, this curry is simple, bursting with flavor and full of nutrition.

Course Dinner, Lunch; Cuisine Indian; Prep Time 10 minutes; Cook Time 18 minutes; Total Time 28 minutes; Servings 3; Calories 419 kcal

## INGREDIENTS:

**For the Tofu**
**For the Spinach Curry**

- **2 tbsp Coconut oil**
- **400 g frozen spinach (thawed)**
- **300 g tofu**
- **1 Tomato**
- **1/2 tsp cumin**
- **200 ml coconut cream**
- **1/2 tsp garam masala**
- **4 cloves garlic**
- **1/2 tsp cayenne pepper**
- **1 tbsp crushed ginger**
- **2 cloves garlic (crushed)**
- **1/4 tsp garam masala**
- **1/4 tsp salt**
- **A pinch of red pepper flakes**

## INSTRUCTIONS:

1. Cut the tofu into 1 inch long strips. Lay down a cotton tea towel and place the tofu on top. Folder the tea towel over onto the tofu and press down to drain the moisture. Do this for a minute or two, rolling the tofu over once to get all the sides.

2. Heat 1 tbsp of coconut oil in a pan on medium high heat and add the tofu. Cook for 10 minutes or until golden brown stirring frequently.

3. In the mean time Add all of the ingredients for the spinach curry into a blender and puree until smooth.

4. Add the garlic to the pan with 1 tbsp of coconut oil and fry for 3 minutes. Add the spinach curry.

5. Cook for a further 5 minutes to let the flavors absorb. Serve immediately.

**Nutritional Information:**

Calories: 419, Fats: 35g, Protein: 15g, Net Carbs: 10g

# Spinach, Avocado and Pumpkin Seed Salad

This refreshing salad is delicious, vegan and keto and full of healthy fats and nutrients. The avocado tastes great, provides some decent calories and is nice and creamy.

Course Dinner, Lunch, Salad; Prep Time 10 minutes; Servings 2; Calories 400 kcal

## INGREDIENTS:

- 2 cups spinach

- 1 cucumber (diced)

- 1 avocado (ripe, diced)

- 1/2 cup pumpkin seeds

- cups cilantro (chopped)

- 1 tbsp lemon juice

- salt and pepper

- 2 tbsp olives (sliced)

- 2 tbsp olive oil

## INSTRUCTIONS:

1. Put spinach, cucumber, avocado, olives and pumpkin seeds in a salad bowl and mix together.

2. Toss with cilantro, lemon juice, olive oil and salt and pepper to taste.

**Recipe Notes**

**This recipe is best served the same day it's made. Although it can survive in the fridge for a day or two - it won't be as fresh!**

**Nutritional Information:**

Calories: 400, Fats: 36g, Protein: 8g, Net Carbs: 6g

# DAILY SNACKS

# Keto Chocolate Protein Shake (Part 1)

Course Drinks; Total Time 5 minutes; Calories 200 kcal; Servings 1.

This keto-vegan beverage is a staple for a veggie lover keto diet.

There are 3 variations intended to give command over what number

of calories you're expending without expanding net carbs. You can include

no coconut oil, 1/8 glass coconut oil or 1/4 container coconut oil.

With 1/4 container coconut oil the smoothie gives 31g of protein

and 670 calories, a significant number of which originate from

medium chain triglycerides which are fats that are effortlessly

utilized by the body for vitality. Contingent upon your calorie

needs, you can change the measure of coconut oil in this beverage.

## INGREDIENTS:

- 1 cup almond milk (unsweetened)
- 2 Scoops Chocolate Protein Powder
- A few ice cubes
- 1/8 - 1/4 cup coconut oil
- A few cubes coffee ice

## INSTRUCTIONS:

1. Pour almond milk into a blender alongside 2 scoops of the protein powder and a couple of ice solid shapes.
2. If you are utilizing coconut oil, place it in a different glass container and microwave for 45 seconds or until melted.
3. Turn the blender on and mix for around 30 seconds.
4. Now while the blend is as yet mixing, gradually empty the coconut oil into the blend. It should take around 10 seconds to pour all the coconut oil. This is critical to permit the coconut oil to completely blend into the smoothie and abstain from bunching or other repulsive surface impacts.
5. Drinks straight away, or put in the ice chest for tomorrow!

**Turn this into a mocha shake**

To make this a mocha shake, just make some dark espresso before hand, to empty it into an ice shape plate and put in freezer. Include these ice cubes to get a decent espresso flavor. Utilize decaf if you need!

# Keto Chocolate Protein Shake (Part 2)

**Recipe Notes:**

This smoothie is a staple in the diet. The nutritional information for the no coconut oil, 1/8 cup and 1/4 cup coconut oil variants have been included. Simply modify it according to your needs!

**Nutritional Information:**

Calories: 200, Fats: 5.5g, Protein: 31g, Net Carbs: 3g

**Nutritional Information with 1/8 Cup Coconut Oil:**

Calories: 425, Fats: 32.8g, Protein: 31g, Net Carbs: 3g

**Nutritional Information with 1/4 Cup Coconut Oil:**

Calories: 671, Fats: 61g, Protein: 30g, Net Carbs: 2g

# Keto Vanilla Protein Shake

This delicious keto-vegan vanilla protein shake offers some assortment to your day by day chocolate shake. Similarly as with the chocolate form there are variations with including 1/8 glass, 1/4 container or no coconut oil. One advantage this one has over the chocolate shake is its net carb tally of 2g rather than 3g.

The ingredients are precisely the equivalent as the chocolate/mocha protein shake, with the exception of you'll utilize the garden of life vanilla protein powder (sport.

**Nutritional Information:**

Calories: 191, Fats: 5.6g, Protein: 32g, Net Carbs: 1g

**Nutritional Information with 1/8 Cup Coconut Oil:**

Calories: 415, Fats: 32.8g, Protein: 31g, Net Carbs: 2g

**Nutritional Information with 1/4 Cup Coconut Oil:**

Calories: 661, Fats: 61g, Proteins: 30g, Net Carbs: 2g

# DESERT

# PUMPKIN SPICE FAT BOMBS

Makes 16 fat bombs / Prep time: 10 minutes, plus 1 hour chilling time

Pumpkin is a great decision for desserts, particularly those that additionally incorporate warm flavors reminiscent of holiday pumpkin pie. Like its vegetable partner, carrots, the brilliant orange tissue of pumpkin shows it is an excellent wellspring of beta-carotene. Pumpkin is additionally high in nutrients An and C and in addition potassium, making this pretty fixing ideal for flushing poisons from your body and battling tumor.

## INGREDIENTS

**½ cup butter, at room temperature**

**1/2 cup cream cheese, at room temperature**

**⅓ 1/3 cup pure pumpkin purée**

**3 tablespoons chopped almonds**

**4 drops liquid stevia**

**½ teaspoon ground cinnamon**

**¼ teaspoon ground nutmeg**

1. Line an 8 square inch container with parchment paper and put aside.
2. In a small bowl, whisk together the butter and cream cheese until very smooth.
3. Add the pumpkin purée and whisk until blended.
4. Stir in the almonds, stevia, cinnamon, and nutmeg.
5. Spoon the pumpkin mixture into the pan. Use a spatula or the back of a spoon to spread it evenly in the pan, then place it in the freezer for about 1 hour.
6. Cut into 16 pieces and store the fat bombs in a tightly sealed container in the freezer until ready to serve.

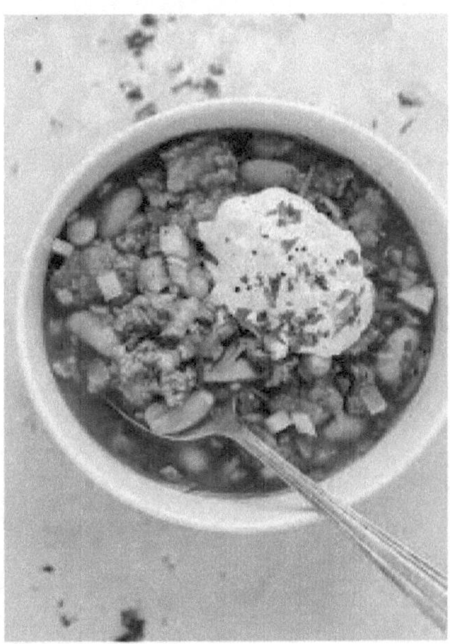

# BLUEBERRY FAT BOMBS

Makes 12 fat bombs / Prep time: 10 minutes, plus 3 hours chilling time

The shade of these fat bombs is a particular blue, which you may discover startling in light of the fact that not very many nourishments are blue. Frozen unsweetened berries will work if fresh are not available or in season: Just thaw the frozen fruit first. On the off chance that your zone has wild blueberries, use these littler berries since they have an altogether more elevated amount of antioxidants against free radicals than grown blueberries.

## INGREDIENTS

½ cup coconut oil, at room temperature

½ cup cream cheese, at room temperature

½ cup blueberries, mashed with a fork

6 drops liquid stevia

Pinch ground nutmeg

## PREPARATIONS

1. Line a smaller scale biscuit tin with paper liners and put aside.

2. In a medium bowl, stir together the coconut oil and cream cheese until well blended.

3. Stir in the blueberries, stevia, and nutmeg until combined.

4. Divide the blueberry mixture into the muffin cups and place the tray in the freezer until set, about 3 hours.

5. Place the fat bombs in an airtight container and store in the freezer until you wish to eat them.

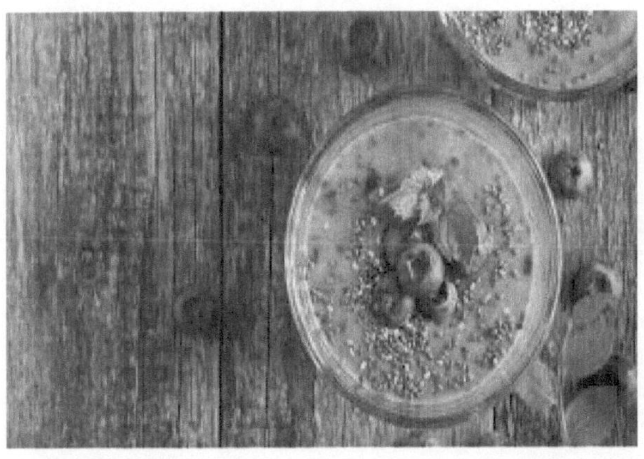

# SPICED-CHOCOLATE FAT BOMBS

Makes 12 fat bombs / Prep time: 10 minutes, plus 15 minutes chilling time / Cook time: 4 minutes

Great quality cocoa powder is an adequate ingredient on the keto-vegan diet, which implies you can in any case appreciate a chocolate pastry and bite when you require a fix. Dull chocolate, for example, cocoa is high in manganese, magnesium, copper, iron, and fiber and also cancer prevention agents, which battle free radicals in the body. Dim chocolate has been found to enable lower to circulatory strain, diminish cholesterol, and enhance intellectual capacity.

## INGREDIENTS

¾ cup coconut oil

¼ cup cocoa powder

¼ cup almond butter

⅛ teaspoon chili powder

3 drops liquid stevia

Line a small scale biscuit tin with paper liners and put aside.

Put a little pan over low warmth and include the coconut oil, cocoa powder, almond spread, stew powder, and stevia. Warmth until the point when the coconut oil is dissolved, at that point race to mix.

Spoon the blend into the biscuit containers and place the tin in the fridge until the point when the bombs are firm, around 15 minutes.

Exchange the glasses to a hermetically sealed holder and store the fat bombs in the cooler until the point when you need to serve them.

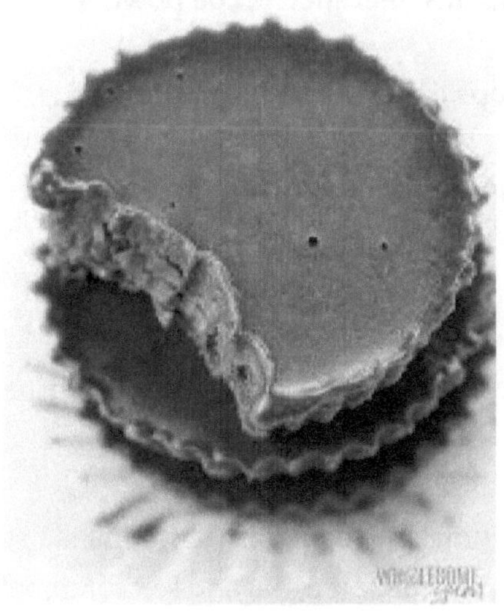

# CHOCOLATE-COCONUT TREATS

Makes 16 treats / Prep time: 10 minutes, plus 30 minutes chilling time / Cook time: 3 minutes

Chocolate and coconut is a flawless combination often found in candy bars and many desserts. If you want a more elegant presentation, omit the coconut in step 3 and roll the semi hardened chocolate mixture into balls instead of spreading it in a pan. Then roll the balls in the shredded coconut and place the treats in the freezer to firm up completely.

## INGREDIENTS

⅓ cup coconut oil

¼ cup unsweetened cocoa powder

4 drops liquid stevia Pinch sea salt

¼ cup shredded unsweetened coconut

## PREPARATIONS

Line a 6-by-6-inch baking dish with parchment paper and set aside.

In a small saucepan over low heat, stir together the coconut oil, cocoa, stevia, and salt for about 3 minutes.

Stir in the coconut and press the mixture into the baking dish.

Place the baking dish in the refrigerator until the mixture is hard, about 30 minutes.

Cut into 16 pieces and store the treats in an airtight container in a cool place.

**PREP TIP** For a more finished look, you can spoon the hot mixture into candy molds instead of a baking dish. Pop the molds in the refrigerator for 30 minutes or until firm and pop the treats out into a cont

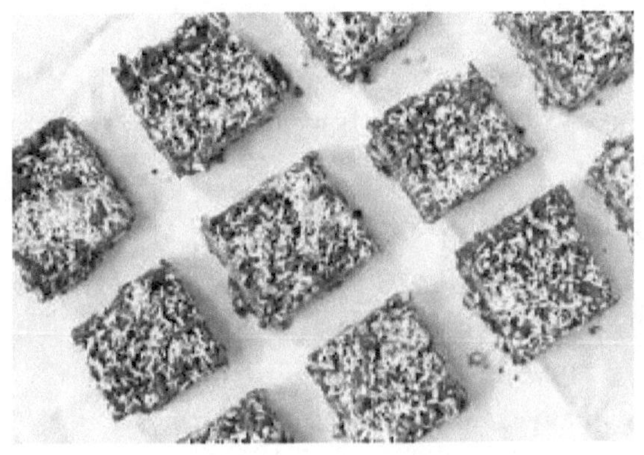

# ALMOND BUTTER FUDGE

Makes 36 pieces / Prep time: 10 minutes, plus 2 hours chilling time

Fudge ought to be smooth and thick with no coarseness or graininess. Since you won't utilize granulated sugar for this treat, the odds of misunderstanding the surface are incredibly diminished. Almond spread is an excellent wellspring of protein, nutrient E, iron, manganese, and fiber. On the off chance that you are not a devotee of this nut margarine, nutty spread or cashew margarine would likewise be flavorful and make the equivalent enticing outcomes.

## INGREDIENTS

**1 cup coconut oil, at room temperature**

**1 cup almond butter**

**¼ Cup heavy cream**

**¼ Pinch sea salt**

**10 Drops liquid stevia**

1. Line a 6-by-6-inch baking dish with parchment paper and set aside.

2. In a medium bowl, whisk together the coconut oil, almond butter, heavy cream, stevia, and salt until very smooth.

3. Spoon the mixture into the baking dish and smooth the top with a spatula.

4. Place the dish in the refrigerator until the fudge is firm, about 2 hours.

5. Cut into 36 pieces and store the fudge in an airtight container in the freezer for up to 2 weeks.

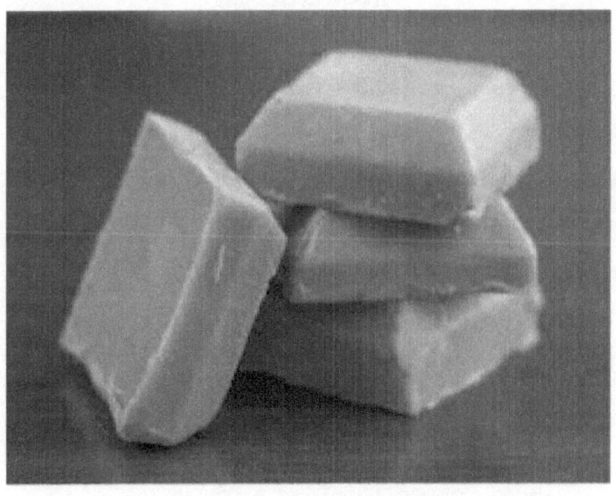

# PEANUT BUTTER MOUSSE

Serves 4 / Prep time: 10 minutes, plus 30 minutes chilling time

Peanut spread is dependably a convenient, delectable sandwich spread, however it is utilized in numerous kinds of dishes everywhere throughout the world, and is extremely sound. Eating nutty spread, even in this delectable sweet, can decrease your danger of malignancy and coronary illness, and help bring down cholesterol levels. Common nutty spread is high in unsaturated fats, protein, fiber, and folate.

## INGREDIENTS

**1 cup heavy (whipping) cream**

**¼ cup natural peanut butter**

**1 teaspoon alcohol-free pure vanilla extract**

**4 drops liquid stevia**

## INSTRUCTION

1. In a medium bowl, beat together the heavy cream, peanut butter, vanilla, and stevia until firm peaks form, about 5 minutes.

2. Spoon the mousse into 4 bowls and place in the refrigerator to chill for 30 minutes.

3. Serve.

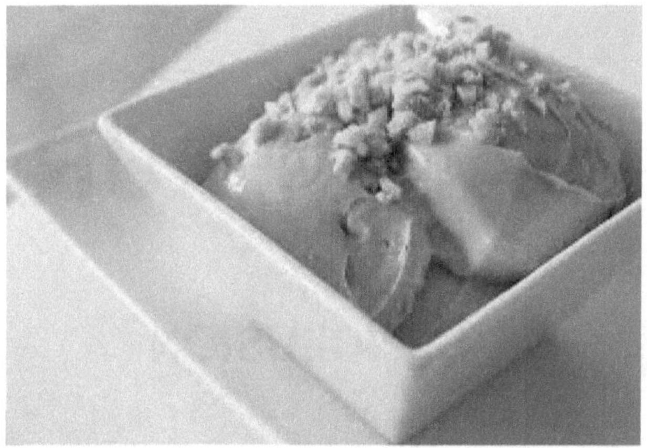

# PART FOUR

## CONCLUSION

# Household Weights and Measurements

## Teaspoons, tablespoons and cups

- 1 metric teaspoon = 5ml/5g
- 1 metric table spoon = 20ml/20g
- 3 tablespoons = 1/4 cup
- 4 tablespoons = 1/3 cup

## Oven Temperatures

| OVEN TEMPERATURES | °C (CELCIUS) | °F (FAHRENHEIT) |
| --- | --- | --- |
| VERY SLOW | 120 | 250 |
| SLOW | 150 | 300 |
| MODERATELY SLOW | 160 | 325 |
| MODERATE | 180 | 350 |
| MODERATELY HOT | 190 | 375 |
| HOT | 200 | 400 |
| VERY HOT | 220-250 | 450-500 |

N.B. When using a fan-forced oven, decrease the oven temperature by 20 ®C.

# ADVICE FOR EATING IN THE RESTAURANT

Getting rid of all culinary temptations is great for eating at home, but what happens when you go out to eat? Staying on a low-carb diet might seem difficult at first, but it can be easy with these few tips and a little bit of practice!

**BREAKFAST**

Skip the bagels, pancakes, Belgian waffles, French toast, or anything of the like. Opt for a side of sausage or ham. Skip the toast and hash browns.

**LUNCH**

Get a salad or garden salad. Use plenty of olive oil and salt (electrolytes). You'll feel great afterward and have plenty of energy to last you until dinner. Carbs are why people get sleepy after lunch. Don't be a victim!

**DINNER**

When ordering a burger, ask to have it wrapped in lettuce. If they're unable to do that, just ask for no bun. If they bring the bun, take the patty and anything else off the bun and put it to the side. Skip the ketchup as well—it's full of sugar. Try mayo, mustard, red pepper sauce, sriracha, or any other low-carb sauce.

At Italian restaurants, skip the pasta and pizza, and order the protein-based dinners. Make sure to request salad or any other low-carb alternatives instead of the usual high-carb sides. If all else fails, just eat the topping off of the pizza and avoid the crust.

With Mexican cuisine, try to get your food in a bowl instead of in a burrito wrap or tortilla. Don't get rice or beans; instead, get extra sour cream and guacamole.

## SIDES

French fries, steak fries, mashed potatoes, baked potatoes, rice, beans, corn on the cob, banana bread, and any other high-carb sides can be replaced with salad, asparagus, broccoli, green beans, or other low-carb vegetables. Most restaurants have some sort of salad for you to choose from. Make sure to always ask and double-check with the waiter or staff.

## DRINKS AND ALCOHOL

Instead of juice or soda, stick to water, tea, and coffee. Use heavy cream or half-and-half instead of milk.

In addition to fat, carbs, and protein, alcohol is also a macronutrient. It provides 7 calories per gram, the second most after fat, which provides 9 calories per gram. It is burned by the body before all the other macronutrients. If you drink too much alcohol, you will slow down your fat-burning process and impede your weight loss, if that is your goal.

If you're ordering alcohol, stay away from any cocktails, as they're all loaded with sugar. Dry or semidry wine has about 3 grams of carbs per glass, and lowcarb beers like Michelob Ultra and Modelo have 3 to 4 grams of carbs per bottle. All pure spirits like vodka, Cognac, brandy, bourbon, whisky, rum, tequila, and gin are zero carbs. As always, drink in moderation, stay safe, and enjoy!

# RESOURCES

## WEBSITES AND BLOGS

**dietdoctor.com**
Diet Doctor is a low-carb-focused site that provides articles and recipes as well as instructional videos and support.

**ketodietapp.com**
Keto Diet App is a keto-only blog and a great resource for science-backed articles and recipes. It also has an app for mobile devices which includes recipes, articles, meal planning, and progress tracking.

**tasteaholics.com**
Tasteaholics is a keto-centric website and resource which provides science-backed articles and recipes.

**authoritynutrition.com/ketogenic-diet-101**
Authority Nutrition is not keto-centric, but it provides many science-backed articles and is a great resource overall.

**alldayidreamaboutfood.com**
One of the oldest low-carb recipe blogs, with more recipes than any other low-carb blog.

**reddit.com/r/keto**
A large community with hundreds of thousands of users, who discuss progress, share cravings, and support each other.

**BOOKS**

Moore, Jimmy, and Eric Westman. *Keto Clarity: Your Definitive Guide to the Benefits of a Low-Carb, High-Fat Diet.* (2014)

Las Vegas, NV: Victory Belt Publishing. A great read and further look into the science behind the keto diet and benefits from eating that diet.

Givens, Sara. *Ketogenic Diet Mistakes: You Wish You Knew.* (2014) Amazon Books. If you hit a weight-loss plateau or are running into any issues, this book can help you break through and reach your goals.

**APPS AND ONLINE TOOLS**

**Keto Macro Calculators:**

**keto-calculator.ankerl.com**
The most detailed and complex.

**ketogains.com/ketogains-calculator**
A simple calculator with no charts and only numbers.

**MyFitnessPal (app)**
A diet and exercise journal which provides meal tracking, calorie and macronutrient tracking, automatic calculation of meal nutrition, exercise tracking and caloric spend, and much more.

www.ingramcontent.com/pod-product-compliance
Lightning Source LLC
Chambersburg PA
CBHW031148250726
48655CB00002B/886

9 781730 963926